Prevent Stroke

Prevent Paralysis That Can

Be Caused By Stroke

Excellent Book

Olatundun Solomon

olatundunsolomon@gmai

l.com

Stroke can be prevented
from occurring. Inside the
head is the brain. The
brain has blood vessels in
it. The brain has arteries
through which blood
flows to nourish the brain.
The brain is used to send
information to the body,
in order to walk, sit, speak
and move the hands. It is

very important to take
care of the brain for the
brain to be healthy. There
are ways by which stroke
can occur. There is
ischemic stroke and also
hemorrhagic stroke.
Ischemic stroke occur
when there is insufficient
blood supply to the brain,
due to the narrowing of
blood vessels while
hemorrhagic stroke is

stroke that occur due to
blood leakage inside the
brain. Hemo- meaning is
blood while -rrhagic
meaning is rupture.
Therefore, hemorrhagic
stroke meaning is sroke
that occurred because of
rupure of blood vessels
inside the brain that led to
blood leakage into the
brain. This makes the
brain not to be well

nourished. And this causes cell death in the brain. To prevent this from happening, the following ways can be used:

(1). Prevent hypertension.

When there is hypertension (high blood pressure), this can make the blood vessels to expand and get weaker. When this occur to the arteries in the brain it can make it to sag and cause aneurysm. When the arteries are very weak, the aneurysm can rupture (burst). When the burst occur it can cause hemorrhagic stroke. It is therefore, very important to prevent hypertension.

Eat vegetables and fruits.
Do exercise. Do not
smoke. Sleep well. Eat
whole grains. Do not drink
alcohol.

(2). Do exercise.

Exercise makes the body
to be healthy. Exercise
can burn fat that may
want to be problem in the
body. Exercise can assist

to burn fat that may want
to narrow blood vessels.
Exercise can make the
heart to be healthy.
Exercise can make the
heart to be healthy.
Exercise can make the
liver to be healthy.
Exercise can make the
body to be healthy.

(3). Do not eat animal fat.

Eating animal fat can

make fat to be

accumulating in the blood

vessels.

Eating animal fat can

make the fat to narrow

blood vessels in the brain.

This can make blood

supply to the brain to be

little. This can make the

brain to be less nourished.

This can cause problem to the brain.

(4). Sleep well.

Sleeping well refreshes the body. This can make the brain to be refreshed. This can make the brain to be healthy.

(5). Take drug according to the prescription correctly for the treatment of sickness.

Taking drug prescription correctly for the treatment of sickness is advisable. Taking overdose of drug can be dangerous to the brain. Taking drug below prescription is not

advisable.

(6). Go to the hospital for

check up.

Going to the hospital for

check up early is advisable.

This can prevent stroke.

This can make a person to

be diagnosed by the

doctor.

(7). Eat vegetables.

Vegetables has vitamins and minerals. This is very good for the body. This can make the brain to be very healthy.

(8). Eat fruits.

Fruits has vitamins and minerals. This can make

the body to be healthy. This can make the brain to be healthy. This can make the brain to have immunity against infections.

(9). Drink enough clean water.

Drinking enough clean water hydrates the body. Drinking enough clean

water can make the blood
to flow freely.

Dehydration can affect
blood flow negatively.
Therefore, hydration can
make the blood to flow
freely to the brain.

Dehydration can make the
blood pressure to be low,
below normal blood
pressure. This can have
negative effect to the
brain.

(10). Do not drink alcohol.

Alcohol drinking can have negative effect to the brain. Alcohol is drying agent. Alcohol drinking can have negative effect to the lungs. It can cause liver cirrhosis. This can cause negative effect in the brain.

(11). Do not smoke.

Smoking can have negative effect to the brain. In the smoke there is carbon monoxide and other harmful gases. This is not beneficial to the brain. What is beneficial

to the brain is oxygen.
Those harmful gases can
have negative effect to
the brain.

(12). Prevent infection of
disease causing
microorganisms.

When disease causing
microorganisms are
prevented. The brain can
be prevented from

disease causing
microorganisms. This can
be done by drinking clean
water, cooking food well
before eating, having bath
with clean water and soap,
having environmental
hygiene and using nose
mask in a dusty
environment.

(13). Take care of the heart.

When the heart is healthy blood can flow well to the brain.

The heart can be taking care of well by not putting too much salt in food. Too much salt in food can make the heart to beat very fast.This can cause chest pain. Do exercise. Exercise can make the heart to be healthy. When the heart is healthy, blood can flow well to the brain to nourish the brain. This can make the brain to be healthy.

(14). Eat protein foods.

Protein food is for growth and development. This food can make the brain to be well developed. The brain need to be well developed in order to function well. Examples of protein foods are titus fish, egg, beans, turkey, chicken and beef.

(15). Eat carbohydrates.

Carbohydrate food gives energy to the body. This makes the brain to be healthy.

Carbohydrate foods are wheat, barley, yam and potatoes.

(16). Wear sit belt when driving car and do not over speed.

Wearing of sit belt when driving car can prevent the head from hitting the wind screen. This can prevent head injury. This can prevent hemorrhagic stroke.

(17). Wear helmet when driving bicycle or motor

bike and do not over

speed. 25

This can prevent accident

and also prevent head

injury. This can prevent

hemorrhagic stroke.

www.ingramcontent.com/pod-product-compliance
Lightning Source LLC
Chambersburg PA
CBHW051240250726
48656CB00003B/1040